I0782147

Methylene Blue For Beginners

Methylene blue, a treatment of malaria, methemoglobinemia, cancer, Alzheimer's disease and aquaculture for the treatment of fish

By

Charles Amelia.

Copyright 2024. All Rights Reserved.

Table of Contents

CHAPTER ONE.

WHAT IS METHYLENE BLUE?

Methylthionine chloride, commonly known as methylene blue, can be prepared as a liquid sedative with a dynamic blue colour. nitrogen sulphur, are amongst its constituents. Methylene blue was created in the 1870s and used as a material dye. In any case, researchers soon discovered its beneficial effects on jungle fever and its antimicrobial and antipsychotic potential.

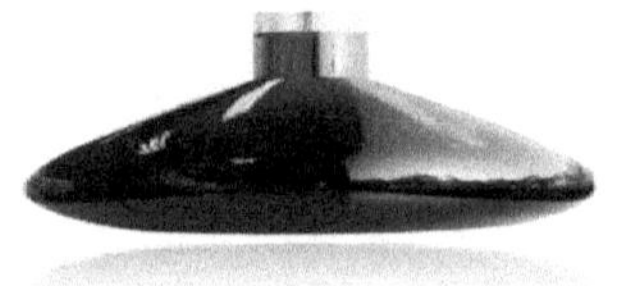

Methylene blue has been used since the 1800s to treat carbon monoxide and cyanide poisoning, as well as methemoglobinemia, a rare disease that affects the blood's ability to carry oxygen. Additionally, methylene blue has neuroprotective properties that help promote a healthy brain. Methylene blue supplementation may additionally promote temperament, memory, focus and fatigue. Methylene blue, a brilliant blue-green natural dye, has its place in the phenothiazine family. It is used for niin (soft vegetable fibres such as jute, flax and hemp) and to a lesser extent for paper, calfskin and coated cotton.

It dyes silk and wool, but these fibres have exceptionally low light fastness. It is also used as a natural dye, in testing sewage for tuberculosis contamination, and as an indicator of chemical oxidation and reduction.

METHYLENE BLUE (METH uh leen bloo), as mentioned above, is used to treat methemoglobinemia. This is often a condition where the blood loses its ability to carry oxygen throughout the body. This guide provides more information about this in the following chapters.

Methylene blue may be a dye that was first created to stain and inactivate certain organisms. It was also one of the main chemotherapy solutions tested in humans, and it to treat intestinal diseases in 1891.

It was superseded by selective strategies but is still used today in histopathology by staining.

Mechanism Of Methylene Blue.

Methylene blue has an oxidized phenothiazine ring framework, in contrast to several other phenothiazine drugs that have a weakened ring structure.

This contrast has important implications for activity and function because it increases the chemical structure point and gives the ring body a positive charge. This allows methylene blue to unexpectedly bind to membranes and intracellular structures. In this case, methylene blue stain can be used again to show layer damage.

One well-established use of methylene blue is as a blood test dye. It unexpectedly targets young blood cells and therefore can be used to describe erythropoiesis (the formation of red blood cells) and age-related breakdown. Drugs with phenothiazine rings, such as methylene blue, are hydrophobic. This can aid in intracellular transport, allowing methylene blue compounds to move within blood cells.

Reduction Agent To Malaria.

The main therapeutic agent of methylene blue was the treatment of jungle fever. It has usually been replaced by other manufactured derivatives capable of treating malaria but has been looked at recently for possible usage again as an antimalarial drug.

Malaria parasites such as Plasmodium falciparum appear to be developing resistance to standard antimalarial drugs. As a result, methylene blue was recovered. Methylene blue was found to have surprising antimalarial effects in cell culture tests. Most critically, creature tests show that the durability of methylene blue is exceptionally muo.

It seems that this could be a practical solution to a problem that is concentrated in the poorest regions of the world. Certain reports of toxic episodes caused by methylene blue therapy should be investigated initially.

These seizures appear to be associated with people who are deficient in G6PD, a critical red blood cell protein. Expanding on malaria parasite control, methylene blue should be useful for a common complication of malaria, methemoglobinemia.

Methemoglobinemia occurs when the haemoglobin bracket is oxidized by iron to the ferrous state. In such a situation oxygen transporting is nearly impossible. The resulting weakness can be fatal. Methylene blue can oxidize NADPH in the methemoglobin formation pathway and is therefore considered potentially useful in preventing this condition.

Protect The Neuro As an Electron Carrier.

It was later shown that methylene blue can be neuroprotective against some cytotoxicity-related diseases such as stroke and Parkinson's disease.

Methylene blue is an electron carrier that allows it to act against jungle fever and methemoglobinemia and is very useful in cytotoxic brain situations because it increases cellular oxygen utilization and decreases anaerobic glycolysis.

Methylene blue can reduce reactive oxygen species (ROS) generation, protect cells from glutamate blockade, attenuate mitochondrial membrane potential depletion, and protect against IAA neurotoxicity, among other beneficial effects.

These benefits are very important in diseases such as Alzheimer's disease, Parkinson's disease and stroke. Coordinated comparisons with antipsychotics such as phenothiazines show that methylene blue has comparable neuroprotective effects, but its components are diverse. Current research indicates that methylene blue is a mitochondria-specific antioxidant that is limited by drugs such as phenothiazines, which are mitochondria-independent free radical scavengers. For previously recorded infections, methylene blue can prevent and control brain damage associated with tumours.

Most alkalines are not mentioned but examples such as ifosfamide are mostly used in the relief of some solid tumours, but they can cause brain damage, which is mitigated by methylene blue. It is not entirely clear how methylene blue prevents brain damage in these cases, but it is likely due to its role in

NADH oxidation and the repair of mitochondrial proteins.

Chemical Composition Of Methylene Blue.
Methylene blue structure.

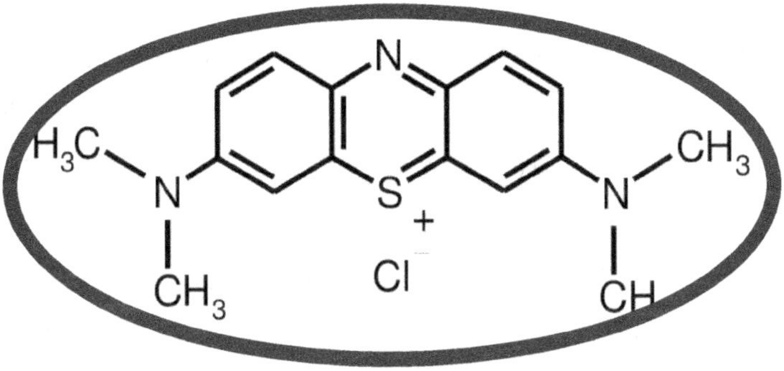

H_3C—N—CH_3 / N—CH_3 / S$^+$ / Cl$^-$ / CH_3 / CH

Methylene blue can be a water solvent, a blue natural dye used as a stain and prescribed medicine that is capable of curing some diseases.

The structure of methylene blue is of no doubt known to be a heterocyclic shape which makes it familiar to know also with an aromatic compound with a central benzene ring and two-sided chains. The dye is cationic, meaning it has an active positive charge and can bond with negatively charged atoms.

The two side chains are critical to the functionality of the dye.

Each side chain has its duties as one side chain is responsible for the dye's ability to bind to DNA, while the other side chain is responsible for the dye's ability to bind to proteins. No side chains can function two jobs at the same time these unique fixtures make methylene blue different from other aromatic substances.

Chemical Formula Of Methylene Blue.

The chemical equation for methylene blue is $C_{16}H_{18}N_3S$. It can be a water-soluble compound that is available as a blue powder or in tablet form. Methylene blue is used as a dye, additive and medicine.

Starting Methylene Blue.

The methylene blue compound can be a water-soluble dye used in various applications, including histological staining and the treatment of methemoglobinemia. Due to the reaction of aniline and sodium hypochlorite, the colour is close to the final colour.

Below are some chemical properties of methylene blue;

- It can be a dull green powder that dissolves in water to a blue solution. Three water atoms per methylene blue unit are in the hydrated form. At 25 °C

(77 °F), water containing 10 g/L methylene blue has a pH of 6

- It can be a commonly used tincture with anti-inflammatory, anti-malarial, anti-inflammatory and anti-cardioprotective effects. effects It functions as a fluorochrome, cholinesterase inhibitor, histological stain, guanylate cyclase inhibitor, and monoamine oxidase inhibitor.
- When some substance is under the oxidation process it synthesises methylene blue.

Physical Properties Of Methylene Blue.

Methylene blue can be a technical organic dye with a blue colour. It can be a cationic dye used as medicine and dye. It is used by physicians or users to ease or remove methemoglobinemia, a disturbing situation in which the blood cannot carry enough oxygen.

It is also used as a dye in various therapeutic trials. Methylene blue can be a water-soluble dye used in various therapeutic tests.

Methylene blue can be a substance that occurs as a crystalline dark green solid or powder and contains a bronze-like lustre. The colour of dead animals in water or liquor is deep blue. In the field of microbiology and chemistry, it is used both as a bacteriological dye and as a marker. Methylene blue can be a dye used as a staining specialist in microscopy, symptomatic procedures and surgery. It is also known as Proveblue, Provable and Urelen Blue.

Below are the physical properties of methylene blue.

- Methylene blue can be a dull green crystalline compound with a mild odour.
- Methylene blue has an atomic mass of 319.0909965 g/mol at 20 °C and a thickness of 1.0 g/ml.

- The melting point of methylene blue is 100-110 °C and at this temperature, it begins to decompose.
- It is soluble in ethanol, chloroform and water and slightly soluble in pyridine but insoluble in ethyl ether.
- It is also soluble in hypochlorite, glycerol, ethanol 2% and acetone 0.5% but insoluble in xylene and oleic acid.
- When heated to the point of destruction, incredibly dangerous nitrogen oxides, sulfur oxides and chlorides are released.

CHAPTER TWO.

HISTORY AND DISCOVERY OF METHYLENE BLUE.

In 1876, Heinrich Caro of Badische Anilin und Pop Fabrik (BASF) synthesized methylene blue (MB) as an aniline-based dye for reddening cotton. A year later, BASF received a German, originally obvious colour (Caro, 1877). Although methylene blue MB (Swiss Blue, Aniline Violet, Methylthionine Hydrochloride, Tetramethylthionine Hydrochloride) accelerated to meet the demands of the materials industry, researchers such as Robert Koch and Paul Ehrlich quickly realized that this was not what it should be.

to maintain different cell structures with different colours, but also mainly to retain and deactivate microbial species. This revelation was in turn based on the testing of these dyes against tropical diseases, and the most prominent candidate for human control was

Methylene Blue MB, which Ehrlich showed in 1891 to be useful in the treatment of malaria. Therefore, methylene blue was the first synthetic compound ever used as a cleaning agent in clinical therapy and the first sterile dye used for therapy.

The use of methylene blue and its subsidiaries has recently been widespread with the introduction of sulfonamides and penicillins in chemotherapy, methylene blue has been a leading compound in studies of various bacterial and viral contaminants and anticancer sedatives, and its contribution has not been specified. . in the phenothiazine family of neuroleptics. In the late 1800s, the growing demand for colours in the next materials industry led to rapid advances in the study of manufactured colours.

One of the most important and obvious results of this progress was the introduction of an endless array of colours into the lifestyle of European cities. The use of primary aniline-based dyes, such as William Perkin's mauve in

1856, increased. everywhere and is authorized to study the use of anilines as dye precursors. For a long time, MB has also been used in human and veterinary medicine for various useful and symptomatic methods, used as a neuroanatomical and bacteriological dye, as thought by an expert on redox stains in biochemistry, as a focus specialist on various cancers. such as melanoma and lung cancer, and as a sterile compound One of the most common clinical applications is methemoglobinemia, whether congenital or drug-induced, mechanical chemicals such as nitrophenols or natural damage such as excess nitrate in well water or cyanide compounds Direct MB.

In the countries that joined in June 2009, 14 clinical trials are included.

explore the clinical utility of Methylene Blue in regions extending from anesthesiology to medications for discouragement and psychosis.

CHAPTER THREE.

METHYLENE BLUE IN TREATMENT OF MALARIA.

Methylene blue has several uses, but the use of methylene blue is that it is used in the treatment of malaria, it is a good antimalarial agent. In this guide, we will briefly explain what malaria is and how methylene blue can be used to treat malaria.

What Is Malaria?

malaria can be an infection caused by a parasite. The virus is transmitted to humans by infected mosquitoes which then causes malaria in humans who are exposed. People with jungle fever usually feel extremely wasted due to high fever and chills. The disease is unprecedented in the temperate zone, but intestinal diseases are still common in tropical and subtropical countries. To reduce contamination from enteric diseases, global welfare programs distribute preventive medicine and insecticide-treated bed nets to protect people from mosquitoes.

The World Health Organization has recommended an enteric vaccine for use in children living in countries with high rates of enteric disease. Protective clothing, bed nets and bug sprays can keep you safe on your trip. In addition, you can take preventive medicines recently, during and after travelling to the risk area. Many jungle fever parasites have developed resistance to the common drugs used to treat the disease.

<u>Symptoms Of Malaria.</u>

Some individuals with jungle fever experience cycles of jungle fever "attacks". An attack usually begins with chills and chills, followed by a high fever, followed by sweating and a return to normal temperature.

Malaria symptoms and side effects usually begin several weeks after being bitten by an infected mosquito. In any case, some jungle fever parasites can rest in your body for up to a year. Some symptoms of malaria are listed below in this guide:

- Chills
- Fever
- Fatigue
- Cough
- Diarrhea
- Headache, etc

Major Causes Of Malaria.

malaria is caused by a single-celled parasite such as Plasmodium. Most often, the parasite infects humans through mosquitoes. Jungle fever spreads when a mosquito transmits the disease after biting an infected person, after which the infected mosquito bites an uninfected person. Jungle fever parasites enter the human bloodstream and travel to the liver. As the parasites develop, they destroy the liver and infect the red blood cells. Some of the ways it spreads are listed below

- **Infected Mosquito:** A mosquito becomes infected by feeding on a person suffering from jungle fever.
- **Transmission of parasites:** If this mosquito bites you in the future, it can transmit intestinal parasites to you.
- **Inside the liver:** When parasites enter your body, they travel to the liver, where some species can live for up to a year.
- **For the circulatory system:** As the parasites develop, they take out your liver and destroy your red blood cells. Usually when individuals develop intestinal diseases.

- **To the next person:** If an uninfected mosquito bites you at this point in the cycle, it becomes infected with dengue parasites and can spread them to other people who have been bitten. Because the parasites that cause jungle fever affect red blood cells, people can also get intestinal diseases from contaminated blood by counting:
- mother to an unborn child
- blood transfusions
- sharing needles used to infuse drugs

<u>Ways To Prevent Malaria.</u>

Mosquitoes are most dynamic between nightfall and daybreak. To ensure yourself from mosquito chomps, you ought to:

- **Don't expose the body's skin:** whatever clothing that can protect the skin is necessary.

- **Apply creepy crawly repellent to skin**: Utilize a creepy crawly repellent enlisted with the Natural Security Organization on any uncovered skin. These incorporate repellents that contain DEET, picaridin, IR3535, oil of lemon eucalyptus (OLE), para-menthane-3,8-diol (PMD) or 2-undecanoate.
Don't utilize a shower directly all over. Don't utilize items with oil of lemon eucalyptus (OLE) or p-Menthane-3,8-diol (PMD) on children under age 3.
- **Apply repellent to clothing:** Showers containing permethrin are secure to apply to clothing.
- **Rest beneath a net:** Bed nets, especially those treated with bug sprays, such as permethrin, help avoid mosquito nibbles while you're resting.

Using Methylene Blue As Anti Agent To Malaria.

Methylene blue was the first directed antimalarial drug created and used to treat all types of jungle fever in the 1800s and early 1900s. Paul Ehrlich and Paul Guttmann recognized methylene blue in 1891 for the treatment of jungle fever. As early as World War I, analysts such as Ehrlich recognized that drugs and dyes worked similarly, based on staining and potentially damaging pathogens.

Soldiers left it in the tropics in the middle of the Pacific War because it has two highlights that make the pee blue or green and the Scalera (white part of the eyes) blue. Methylene blue MB acted synergistically with artemisinin derivatives in preliminary assays and had a significant effect on the reduction of P-gametocytes. falciparum. As a result, methylene blue has been recognized as a potential adjunct in artemisinin-based combination therapy (ACT), especially when eradication is the ultimate goal. It was then widely used against many pests and all subtypes of jungle fever, especially jungle fever, which did not respond well to quinine treatment.

Methylene blue is FDA-approved and is one of the safest medications. Because of its low price, its use as an antimalarial drug has attracted attention, which has recently resurfaced. Many clinical trials are underway to find an acceptable combination for this sedative.

Component Of Methylene Blue Against Malaria Sickness.

The antimalarial activity of methylene blue has been associated with antioxidant responses that specifically target glutathione reductase, a key protein in the life cycle of P. falciparum. Methylene blue reduces parasite overlap in the late trophozoite stage when haemoglobin absorption is severe; this decrease in parasite proliferation coincides with a change in the plasmodial GR peak during the 24th hour of the intraerythrocytic cycle. Methylene blue reaches maximum plasma levels in humans 1-2 hours after oral ingestion of 100 mg. It has a plasma half-life of approximately 5-6.5 hours and a moderate renal excretion rate of nearly 20-30%.

CHAPTER FOUR.

METHEMOGLOBINEMIA.

In the previous chapter of this book, we saw the concept of malaria and how methylene blue can be used as a treatment, so in this chapter, we will now look at methemoglobinemia and the possible ways methylene blue can help in treatment.

The Concept Of Methemoglobinemia And Treatment Using Methylene Blue.

What Is Methemoglobinemia?:

Methemoglobinemia (MetHb) can be an extremely rare blood disorder, sometimes called "blue baby syndrome," that affects how red blood cells carry oxygen to cells and tissues. People can develop the disease, but MetHb usually occurs when people use certain solutions or recreational drugs or are exposed to certain chemicals. Most people with methemoglobinemia have some level of cyanosis, which turns the nail beds, tongue, lips, and skin a certain light blue or purple shade. Red blood cells regularly carry oxygen throughout the body. Red blood cells depend on the protein haemoglobin to transport oxygen. In MetHb, an inherited change turns haemoglobin into methemoglobin. Methemoglobin does not carry oxygen. Without adequate blood oxygenation, the amount of oxygen in the blood forms cyanosis.

Symptoms Of Methemoglobinemia:

Side effects vary depending on the type of condition. Most people with MetHb develop the condition because they take certain painkillers or recreational drugs or are exposed to certain toxic substances. This is often due to methemoglobinemia and side effects can include:

- fatigue
- weakness
- headache
- pale pale skin
- sickness and vomiting.
- Extraordinary lethargy, slurred speech and moderate reflexes: These are signs of the central nervous system.
- Loss of consciousness or wild jerky movements: These are signs of seizures.
- Rapid breathing, increased heart rate and disorientation: These are signs of metabolic acidosis. of.

congenital symptoms include:

Congenital methemoglobinemia is extremely rare and only a few cases have been recorded worldwide. Based on this information, healthcare providers have defined three types of congenital methemoglobinemia — type 1, type 2, and haemoglobin M (HbM) disease. People with haemoglobin infection regularly have cyanosis but are otherwise healthy. People with category 1 MetHb have cyanosis but sometimes have other repair problems. On the other hand, babies born with Sort 2 MetHb often develop severe neurological problems before 9 months and sometimes live beyond the earliest stage.

Causes Of Methemoglobinemia.

Individuals acquire or develop this condition through the use of certain drugs, recreational drugs, or exposure to certain toxins. Less often, people suffer from this form of the condition. People can also develop methemoglobinemia when exposed to nitrates used in some medications, nitrites (chemicals used in food additives and well water), and certain horticultural herbicides. People who use recreational drugs such as amyl nitrite (poppers), nitrous oxide (rim gas), and local anaesthetics or pain relievers used to "cut" cocaine are more likely to develop life-threatening medical problems due to abnormally high methemoglobin levels. Hereditary, other causes of methemoglobinemia may include Two different inherited changes that cause congenital MetHb. Haemoglobin M disease occurs when certain types of haemoglobin M change.

Intrinsic methemoglobinemia is an autosomal recessive disorder, which means that both parents have inherited changes that they pass on to their organic children.

Haemoglobin M disease is autosomal, which means that one of the parents passes the hereditary change on to their organic children.

Test And Diagnosis Of Methemoglobinemia.

Diagnostic feature: Healthcare providers diagnose this condition through a thorough medical history and physical examination. They may ask about individuals who show signs of acquired MetHb if they are taking any medications or if they have been exposed to any harmful substances. Healthcare providers may perform certain testing procedures:

- Blood tests: People with this condition often have dull brown blood in their veins. A dark brown colour can be a sign that the blood in the vessel does not carry oxygen.
- MetHb assessment: Healthcare providers measure the level of methemoglobin in your blood.
- Genotyping: most physicians carry out hereditary checks on patients to ascertain if there is any hereditary transmission of methemoglobinemia. Using genotyping, healthcare providers identify the type of disease.
- Haemoglobin electrophoresis: This process is often used by most healthcare providers to test the level of haemoglobin in your red blood cells. They can use this test to diagnose HbM.

Treatment Of Methemoglobinemia.

Treatment changes are based only on methemoglobinemia. For example, a child suffering from a different type of illness needs exceptionally different treatment than the one causing the illness, because he was exposed to harmful substances If so, healthcare providers can use post-treatment solutions to lower methemoglobin levels:

- Methylene blue
- Vitamins C and B2

Throughout this chapter, we will look at how methylene blue is used to treat methemoglobinemia, but depending on the circumstances, obtained methemoglobinemia can be a restorative crisis that requires urgent treatment, such as intravenous fluids and oxygen.

Treatment Of Metheglobinemia Using Methylene Blue.

Methylene blue is known for its oxidizing properties and it is because of this property that it works as a treatment for methemoglobinemia. Methylene blue oxidizes NADPH and becomes leuco methylene blue. In this step, leu-comethylene blue oxidizes methemoglobin and converts it to haemoglobin.

Methylene blue returns the haemoglobin clamp to its normal (reduced) oxygen-carrying state. Usually ended with a fictitious electron acceptorMethylene blue treatment does not work for those with glucose-6-phosphate dehydrogenase (G6PD) deficiency, because G6PD can be a key compound in NADPH production, and if sufficient NADPH is not achieved controlled methylene. blue will not change. An excess of unreduced methylene blue can oxidize the haemoglobin itself, causing more methemoglobin to be produced. Providing demonstrable evidence of disease and treatment is initiated when warranted (especially in acquired methemoglobinemia), which is essential in the management of methemoglobinemia.

At the same time, it may be important to initiate extensive, regularly disturbing tests to rule out cardiac and respiratory problems that lead to regular clinical use comparable to cyanosis. Methylene blue USP is given into a vein by IV.

This infusion is given by a doctor. The total duration of intravenous implantation can last up to 30 minutes. It is administered by dosing 1-2 mg/kg as a 1% solution in IV saline over 3-5 minutes. Blood pressure, oxygen levels, kidney function, and other important factors are constantly monitored. Your blood will also be tested so your specialist can assess whether the medicine is working. You may need one dose of methylene blue. If you need a moment of measurement, it can be given one hour after the pre-selection. Methylene blue will almost certainly make you pee or turn your face blue or green. In general, the common side effects of the drug do not have negative results. This effect, whatever it may be, can produce unexpected results in any urinalysis. Starting treatment involves regulating supplemental oxygen and removing the troublesome oxygen chemicals.

The first-line treatment is intravenous (IV) methylene blue. MetHb levels should be rechecked after MB therapy. MB should not be administered to patients with impaired glucose-6-phosphate dehydrogenase (G6PD) because MB-induced MetHb reduction is dependent on NADPH produced by G6PD (hemolysis). Caustic ascorbic acid (2 mg/kg) is an alternative treatment for these people.

 In patients with extreme methemoglobinemia who are refractory to methylene blue or cannot be treated with methylene blue, commercial transfusion and oxygen therapy are second-line options.

How To Prevent Methemoglobinemia.

Individuals who develop some form of this condition should avoid harmful substances such as pesticides, some drugs, and most anaesthetics that cause methemoglobin levels to rise. If you are at risk for this condition, ask your doctor about which substances and medications you should avoid. People who use recreational drugs such as amyl nitrite or cocaine are at greater risk of methemoglobinemia. If you are taking these medications and want help to quit smoking, talk to your doctor about possible medications or programs that may help you.

CHAPTER FIVE.

CANCER AND TREATMENT OF CANCER USING METHYLENE BLUE.

Cancer can be a large group of infections with one thing in common: they all occur when normal cells become cancer cells that multiply and spread. Cancer starts when some quality or some characteristics change and form cancer cells. These cells form cancerous tumours or tumours. Cancer cells can break free from tumours by using your lymph tissue or circulatory system to travel to other areas of your body. (Healthcare providers call this metastasis.)In this case, a tumour in the chest can spread to the lungs, making it difficult to breathe. In some types of blood cancer, abnormal cells in your bone marrow produce irregular blood cells that reproduce wildly. In the long run, the irregular cells crowd out the typical blood cells.

Some Common Cancer:

- **Breast cancer:** cancer is nothing new but one that's familiar is no other than breast cancer. It mainly affects women and individuals AFAB. However, almost 1% of all breast cancers affect men and people with AMAB.
- **Lung cancer:** Lung cancer is the most common cancer today. small and non-small cell lung cancer are the two kinds as provided in this guide.
- **Prostate cancer:** One in nine men and people with AMAB suffer from this cancer.
- **Colon cancer:** Colon cancer and rectal cancer affect different parts of the body related to the stomach.

- Blood cancers: the blood has its cancer and we can't mention any without telling you about Leukemia and lymphoma

Symptoms Of Cancer:

Cancer can be a complicated disease. Cancer can be without symptoms for a long time. Sometimes cancer can cause telltale signs that become more unfortunate at an extraordinary rate. Many cancer symptoms occur after other less real diseases. It's not cruel to get certain signs that you have cancer. In general, you should talk to your doctor whenever you notice a change in your body that lasts more than two weeks.

Some of the symptoms are:

- Constant fatigue.
- Inexplicable on my scale.
- Unrelenting agony.
- Fever usually occurs at night.

- Skin changes, especially moles that change shape and size or modern moles. Untreated, cured cancer can cause additional side effects, including Lumps or lumps under the skin that won't go away.
- Difficulty breathing.
- Feel free to get bruised or die.
- Difficulty swallowing.
-

Diagnosis And Test Of Cancer:

Healthcare providers begin the diagnosis of cancer with a thorough physical examination. They ask you to describe your references. They may ask about almost any medical history in your family. They may also take a sample after the tests:

- Biopsies.
- Blood tests.
- Image tests.

Biopsies

A biopsy may be a procedure that healthcare providers use to obtain cells, tissue, fluid, or growth material that they can see under a magnifying glass. There are several types of biopsies:

- **Needle biopsy**: This test may be called fine needle aspiration or fine needle biopsy. Needle biopsies are routinely performed to screen for breast cancer, thyroid cancer, or lymph node cancer.
- **Skin biopsy**: Healthcare providers remove a small sample of your skin to analyze for skin cancer.
- **Bone marrow biopsy:** Health care providers do a small test of the bone marrow so they can test for signs of disease and calculate the amount of cancer in your bone marrow.
- **Endoscopic or laparoscopic biopsy**: These biopsies use an endoscope or laparoscope to see inside your body. In

both strategies, a small incision is made in your skin and the instrument is inserted. An endoscope can be a thin, flexible tube with a camera at the end and a cutting device next to it to remove the test. The laparoscope has a somewhat diverse field of application.

- **Excisional or excisional biopsy:** In these open biopsies, a specialist cuts into your body and either the entire tumour is removed (excisional biopsy) or part of the tumour is evacuated (incisional biopsy) for testing or treatment.

- **Perioperative biopsy:** This test may be called a fixed segment biopsy. This biopsy is done while another method is being used. Your tissue will be evacuated and sampled. It happens shortly after the procedure, so if you want treatment, you can start it right away.

Blood tests

Blood tests for cancer may include:

- **Complete blood count (CBC):** A CBC test measures and checks your blood cells.
- **Tumor markers:** Tumor markers are substances secreted by cancer cells or normal cells in response to cancer cells.
- **Blood protein tests:** Healthcare providers use a probe called electrophoresis to measure immunoglobulins. The immune system responds to certain cancers by releasing immunoglobulins.
- **Tests for circulating tumour cells:** Cancerous tumours can shed cells. Tumor cell tracking has implications for healthcare providers when screening for cancer activity.

Imaging tests Imaging tests may include:

- **Computed tomography (CT) scan:** CT checks the area of the cancer and the effect on organs and bones.
- **X-rays:** X-rays use a safe amount of radiation to create images of your bones and sensitive tissues.
- **Positron Emission Test (PET) Filter:** PET creates images of your working organs and tissues. Healthcare providers can use this test to detect early signs of cancer.
- **Ultrasound:** An ultrasound uses high-intensity sound waves that seem to cut apart the inside of your body.
- **Excited Magnetic Resonance Imaging (MRI):** MRIs use a huge magnet, radio waves, and a computer to take pictures of your organs and other internal parts of your body.

Iodometaidobenzylguanidine (MIGB): This nuclear imaging test makes a difference in distinguishing between cancers, including carcinoid tumors, and neuroblastoma. disappeared. It happens shortly after the strategy, so if you want treatment, you can start it right away.

- **Hereditary testing**: cancer can occur when one trait changes or several traits that work together change. Analysts have identified more than 400 properties related to cancer treatment. Individuals who acquire these traits from their organic guardians may be more likely to develop cancer. Healthcare providers may order tests for hereditary cancer if you have an acquired form of cancer. They can also do genetic testing to make treatments that target certain characteristics of the cancer. They use tests to conclude. They will split a number or arrange your conclusion.

Let's look at some stages of cancer: Most cancers have four stages. The specific stage is determined by many different variables, including the grade and size of the tumour:

- **Stage I:** The cancer is localized to a small area and has not spread to lymph nodes or other tissues.
- **Arrange II:** The cancer has progressed but has not spread.
- **Organization III:** The cancer has grown and may have spread to lymph nodes or other tissues.
- **Stage IV:** This arrangement is also called metastatic or advanced cancer.

  Although stages 1 to 4 are the most common, stage 0 also exists. This most specific stage describes cancer that is still localized to the area where it started. Precancerous can be treated even when it is already in the body thus, said by most healthcare providers.

<u>Treatment Of Cancer.</u>

Healthcare providers may use some different medications, sometimes combining medications depending on the circumstances. The most common anti-cancer treatments are:

- **Chemotherapy:** Chemotherapy is one of the most common anti-cancer treatments. It uses drugs that can destroy cancer cells. You will receive chemotherapy in pill form or intravenously (through a needle into a vein). In some cases, providers may coordinate chemotherapy in a specific affected area.
- **Radiotherapy:** This treatment kills cancer cells with high doses of radiation. Your doctor may combine radiation therapy with chemotherapy.
- **Surgery:** Cancers that have not spread can be evacuated through surgery. Your doctor can recommend treatment. This

treatment combines surgery with chemotherapy or radiation to shrink the tumour before surgery or to kill any remaining cancer cells after surgery.

- **Hormone therapy:** Sometimes providers recommend hormones that produce other cancer hormones.
- **Organic Reaction Transformation Treatment:** This treatment improves your safety and improves its performance.
- **Cancer immunotherapy:** Immunotherapy can be a cancer treatment that locks in your immune system to fight the disease. The treatment can be called naturopathy.
- **Targeted cancer therapy:** Targeted cancer therapy can target inherited changes or transformations that turn normal cells into cancer cells.
- **Bone marrow transplant:** A treatment called a stem cell transplant replaces damaged stem cells with healthy ones.

An autologous transplant uses your healthy stem cells. An allogeneic transplant uses stem cells donated by another person.

Methylene Blue And Cancer Treatment.

Methylene blue, a manufactured dye, has been used in various therapeutic applications for over a century. Be that as it may, subsequent reflections have shed hitherto untapped light on its potential as an anti-cancer treatment. In this guide, we look at the properties of methylene blue, and its potential role in cancer treatment, Additionally, we explore how the Mending Cancer Center, led by Dr. Leigh Erin Connealy, incorporates methylene blue into their treatment plans for cancer patients. Methylene blue can be an engineered compound with a deep blue colour that has been used for various therapeutic purposes. Created as a dye for materials, it was later found to have anti-malarial properties and was used to treat intestinal ailments during the First World War. Since then, methylene blue has been used as an antibacterial specialist and to treat several diseases. , which may include Alzheimer's disease, and methemoglobinemia carbon monoxide Recently, studies have explored the potential of methylene blue in cancer treatment.

It is believed that methylene blue can be useful in preventing tumour development and reducing the spread of cancer cells. It is accepted that it inhibits the production of vitality in cancer cells, which can lead to cell migration. The centre focuses on the use of methylene blue in cancer treatment, which has been shown to have critical potential in controlling and promoting the development of tumours with beneficial results. Methylene blue is an FDA-approved drug that has been used for decades in various therapeutic settings and has been used to treat conditions such as methemoglobinemia and as a staining agent during surgical strategies. Subsequent studies further highlighted its potential in cancer treatment, as it can inhibit cancer development and promote cancer cell migration.

At the Cancer Recovery Center, methylene blue is used as part of a comprehensive treatment plan that includes multiple modalities and treatments tailored to each patient's needs.

This personalized approach to treatment ensures that each understanding receives the best possible feasible and appropriate care. Combining methylene blue with treatment at a cancer centre involves several steps.

Initially, the calm undergoes a careful restorative evaluation and symptom tests to decide the type and order of cancer. At that time, the expert group of the centre plans an individualized treatment plan, where methylene blue focuses on anti-cancer treatment. Methylene blue is often administered intravenously in a carefully controlled environment to ensure ideal dosage and safety. Depending on certain types of cancer and treatment needs, this insight can also be embraced in the methylene blue formulation. Methylene blue can be a powerful tool in the fight against cancer, whether used alone or in combination with other targeted anticancer drugs.

The Cancer Recovery Center is committed to staying at the forefront of this energizing research and advancing its application in the lives of cancer patients.

Importance Of Methylene Blue In Cancer Treatment.

Cancer cells have no hiding place for methylene blue when introduced hence its crucial role in cancer treatment is very beneficial. Not at all like conventional chemotherapy drugs, which can damage both solid cells and cancer cells, methylene blue appears to target cancer cells while leaving healthy cells unharmed. It reduces the side effects of chemotherapy, such as hair loss and disease. Methylene blue also appears to improve the cost-effectiveness of other cancer treatments, such as radiation therapy. By sensitizing cancer cells to radiation, methylene blue can help promote outcomes and reduce the risk of cancer recurrence.

Methylene Blue Acting As A Cancer Therapy.

Methylene blue has cancer treatment potential due to its ability to target cancer cells and prevent the development of tumours. Later, it is considered and clinical trials have investigated its applicability in the treatment of various cancers, including breast, prostate and bladder cancer. One of how methylene blue exerts its anticancer effects is by focusing on the powerhouse of cancer cells.

 Methylene blue has been found to disrupt the electron transport chain in cancer cell mitochondria, which reduces ATP production and ultimately causes cancer cell apoptosis. In one study, a combination of methylene blue and radiation therapy was found to be more effective than either treatment alone in preventing tumour development in mice with breast cancer.

Dr Leigh Erin Connealy provides information that methylene blue is mostly used and the centre never ceases to promote it out. The centre uses a comprehensive approach that combines different categories to meet the individual needs of each understanding. The role of methylene blue in preventing the development of tumours makes it a potentially effective extension of the centre's focused cancer treatment.

Methylene Blue As A Potential Cancer Prevention Agent.

Methylene blue has been identified as a potential anticancer agent. Its antioxidant and anti-inflammatory properties reduce the risk of cancer. As discussed later, methylene blue can help prevent cancer by slowing the growth of cancer cells and reducing the number of changes that lead to cancer.

Methylene blue can also be used in the early site and stage of cancer. Research suggests that methylene blue could be used to differentiate cancer cells, making it less demanding for specialists to analyze the infection in its early stages. Once identified, methylene blue can be used as part of a comprehensive regimen designed to target and prevent tumour development.

Future Role Of Methylene Blue For Cancer Treatment.

When it comes to researching the potential of methylene blue in cancer treatment, there is promising evidence that this compound can have significant effects on cancer cells.

Since then, it has been found that methylene blue can prevent the development of tumours in various cancers, including breast, colon and lung cancer. One way methylene blue affects cancer cells is by triggering apoptosis, or programmed cell death. This can be crucial because cancer cells are known for their ability to avoid apoptosis and grow and multiply wildly. By activating apoptosis, methylene blue can target and eliminate cancer cells. Expanding on its role in initiating apoptosis, methylene blue has also been shown to have antioxidant and anti-inflammatory properties. These properties can help protect the vocal cords from damage caused by oxidation and deterioration, which is known to promote cancer healing and movement. Although much research remains to be done, the long-term use of methylene blue in cancer treatment appears promising.

CHAPTER SIX.

ALZHEIMERS DISEASE USING METHYLENE BLUE AS TREATMENT.

What Is Alzheimer's Disease:

Alzheimer's disease can be a brain disorder that gets worse over time. It is characterized by changes in the brain that lead to the storage of certain proteins. Alzheimer's causes the brain to contract in abnormal order. Alzheimer's disease is the most common cause of dementia, a progressive decline in memory, behaviour and social skills. approximately 55 million people worldwide with dementia, 60 to 70 percent have Alzheimer's disease. Early signs of the condition include ignoring subsequent events or conversations. Over time, this develops into real memory problems and trouble with normal tasks. Resources can improve or slow down the movement of side effects. Programs and administrations can assist in supporting people with the disease and their caregivers. No treatment cures Alzheimer's disease. In advanced stages, severe brain dysfunction can lead to dehydration, poor health or pollution. These complications can lead to death.

Symptoms Of Alzheimer's.

Memory loss is a major side effect of Alzheimer's disease. Early signs include difficulty remembering subsequent events or conversations. But memory deteriorates and other side effects appear as the infection progresses. At first, the infected may be aware that he has trouble remembering things and thinking clearly. If symptoms become more severe, a family member or partner may become more aware of problems. Brain changes associated with Alzheimer's cause the following disorders:

Memory: Everyone has memory problems at some point, but Alzheimer's is permanent and gets worse. Alzheimer's disease can result in memory loss which may decline overall daily performance by ignoring conversations, agreements, or events.

- Lose things and often put them in meaningless places.
- Enter places they knew. In the long run, ignore the names and shared objects of family members.
- You have trouble finding the right words for things, communicating your thoughts, or participating in conversations.
- Repeat the articulations and questions over and over.
- **Reasoning and thinking:** Alzheimer's disease causes difficulty concentrating and reasoning, especially unique

concepts such as numbers. Doing more than one task at a time is especially difficult. Keeping up with accounts, adjusting checks and paying bills on time can be difficult. In the long term, a person with Alzheimer's disease may not be able to recognize and negotiate numbers.

- **Judgments and choices:** Alzheimer's disease impairs the ability to make rational choices and decisions under normal circumstances. For example, a person may make poor choices in a social setting or wear a dress outside the basic climate. Frequently asked questions can be more difficult to answer. For example, a person may not know how to deal with food burning on the stove or options while driving.
- **Organization and Completion of Identifiable Tasks:** Design exercises that require you to go through the steps of organizing a battle. This could include

organizing and cooking dinner or playing your favourite song. In the long term, people with advanced Alzheimer's disease don't worry about how to take care of basic things like getting dressed and showering.

- **Changes in identity and behaviour:** Brain changes associated with Alzheimer's disease can affect attitudes and behaviour. Problems can include the following factors:
- Exciting unhappiness in exercises.
- Social withdrawal.
- Depression.
- Anger or hostility.
- Postural fluctuations.
- Suspicion of others.
- Changes in inclination to rest.
- Wandering.
- Prevents bad luck.
- Dreams are like accepting that something is stolen.

- **Preserved skills:** Despite significant changes in memory and skills, individuals with Alzheimer's disease may retain some skills as symptoms become more severe. Protected skills may include reading or tuning books, telling stories, sharing memories, singing, setting music, moving, drawing or creating. These abilities can be protected longer because they are controlled by parts of the brain that are later affected by the infection. Causes of Alzheimer's disease. the result of the cause of this disease may not be fully comprehended. But at baseline, the brain's proteins cannot function normally. It interrupts the activity of brain cells, also called neurons and triggers opportunities. Neurons are damaged and lose connection with each other. Finally, the bucket was kicked. Scientists agree that most people develop Alzheimer's because of genetics, lifestyle and natural factors that affect the brain over time. In less than 1 per cent of cases, Alzheimer's disease is caused by certain inherited changes that almost guarantee that a person will develop the disease. In such cases, the infection usually begins in middle age. In the case of the last primary indications, the development of the infection begins for a long time. The deficits usually begin in the area of the brain that controls memory.

The neuronal accident spreads somewhat unexpectedly to other areas of the brain. In the late stages of the disease, the brain is significantly reduced. Analysts trying to figure out the cause of Alzheimer's disease are focusing on a cross-section of two proteins:

- **Tangle:** Tau proteins are part of the inner spine of the brain cell and the transport backbone for transporting nutrients and other vital materials. Cells disrupt the transport framework and damage cells.

- **Plaques:** beta-amyloid can be part of a larger protein. When these parts accumulate, they have a toxic effect on neurons and disrupt communication between brain cells. These clumps form larger deposits called amyloid plaques, which also contain other cellular rafts and jetsam.

Applying Methylene Blue As Treatment Of Alzheimer's Diseases:

Methylene blue can be an excellent treatment for Alzheimer's disease. Methylene blue can make progress on the side effects of Alzheimer's disease by combining various neuro-fibrillary tangles caused by the aggregation of a protein called Tau in brain neurons. The clinical side effects of Alzheimer's disease are more related to Tau protein than to amyloid plaques. Methylene blue can impair tau organization through its effects on mitochondria, which should delay and/or delay clinical signs of Alzheimer's disease. Methylene blue may be an excellent treatment for Alzheimer's disease. Methylene blue can progress on Alzheimer's symptoms by combining different ones. The neurological effects of Alzheimer's disease include amyloid plaques (aggregates of amyloid protein in the grey matter of the brain) and neurofibrillary tangles. Neurofibrillary tangles are caused by the accumulation of a protein in the brain called Tau interneurons. The clinical symptoms of Alzheimer's disease are more related to Tau protein than to amyloid plaques. Methylene blue can impair tau organization through its effects on mitochondria, which should promote and/or delay clinical signs of Alzheimer's disease.

Methylene Blue In Treating Covid 19.

Methylene blue also has a guarantee in the treatment of long-term indications of COVID-19. Methylene blue has anti-inflammatory properties against inflammatory cytokines that are released during the immune response to COVID-19 contamination. Its anti-inflammatory effect appears to be by inhibiting the NLRP3 inflammasome complexes on macrophages, which dramatically reduces the number of inflammatory cytokines that can cause damage to vital organs.

COVID can cause cells to stress and lead to the organization of free radicals through the oxidative acceleration of mitochondria, the heart of the life force arrangement. The placement of free radicals can cause the questionable irritation often seen in patients with COVID. In addition, methylene blue reduces oxidative stress caused by free radical placement, promoting mitochondrial fitness. This should reduce some of the incessant anger that often plagues many COVID patients. Methylene blue can additionally offer help to people who suffer from constant torment, especially by its definition, verbal flushing. Methylene blue can reduce torture through various components. Adjuvant methylene blue seems to affect different levels of nociceptive (pain receptors). In addition, methylene blue has an advantage over other oral rinses used in the treatment of torture because many oral rinses used in torture have the side effect of local anaesthesia, which manifests itself as numbness in the mouth.

This leads to continued nonadherence to medication because oral mortality can change the taste of dinner. In any case, methylene blue does not cause local anaesthesia, so silence does not meet the feeling of death in the mouth. This is likely to result in a better understanding of compliance in patients using methylene blue, unlike other verbal washes used for torture. This makes methylene blue an excellent choice for patients who endure unrelenting agony. Methylene blue can be mixed in various dosage forms, but the most common is the capsule body. According to the literature, the normal dose of methylene blue is 0.5-4mg/kg. Anything above 5 mg/kg is considered harmful. Moo Measurements Methylene blue has the main beneficial effect and is usually administered at 10-30 mg/day. However, the optimal dosage is highly individualized and each patient should work with their healthcare provider to find the right measurements for them. Additionally, it is important to distinguish between the USP grade of methylene blue and other grades. USP allows contamination of < 0.5% in the methylene blue definition. Reducing agents may contain potentially toxic metals such as arsenic, mercury, lead, etc. In any case, multiple mechanical determinations of methylene blue can result in a reduction of more than 10%. It is dangerous if these pollutants contain potentially harmful substances. Reductions are also another reason methylene blue measurement is preferred over larger measurements, as the risk of reduction increases as the methylene blue measurement increases. The mixing of methylene blue should be defined based on the USP overview. Although MB is an ancient medicine, it can be a success in the treatment of various infections. People with many diseases can be lighter and longer with methylene blue.

<u>Risky Factors To Be Considered:</u>

- **Down syndrome as a risk factor:** It is usually associated with three duplicates of chromosome 21. Chromosome 21 is a trait associated with the production of a protein that leads to the formation of beta-amyloid. Beta-amyloid particles can end up in the brain as plaques. Side effects usually occur 10 to 20 times earlier in people with Down syndrome than in the general population.

- **Age**: Increasing age is the most important known risk factor for Alzheimer's disease. But as you become more experienced, the possibility of creating it increases. It is estimated that four contemporary analyses were performed per thousand 65-74-year-olds each year. Among those aged 75-84, there were 32 contemporary analyses per 1,000 people. There were 76 contemporary analyses per 1,000 people aged 85 and over.

- **Family history and inherited traits**: The chance of developing Alzheimer's disease is slightly higher if a first-degree relative - your parent or relative - has the disease. How familial characteristics affect risk is largely unexplained, and heritable variables are likely to be complex. Much better; Much better; developed Stronger; Improved A much better captured hereditary indicator could be the quality of apolipoprotein E (APOE). A high APOE e4 frame increases the risk of Alzheimer's disease. Almost 25-30% of the population is APOE e4. But not everyone who has such a high-quality frame causes disease. Researchers have found rare changes in three traits that essentially guarantee that a person with one of them will develop Alzheimer's disease. However, these changes occur in less than 1 per cent of people with Alzheimer's disease.

- **Gender:** Generally there are more women because they live longer than men.

- **Mild Cognitive Impairment:** A person with mild Cognitive Impairment (MCI) has a decline in memory or other cognitive abilities that is more pronounced than normal for the person's age. However, the bill does not prevent a person from functioning in social or work situations. However, people with MCI are at significant risk of developing dementia. If MCI primarily affects memory, the condition is more likely to progress to Alzheimer's dementia. The MCI finding gives people the opportunity to focus more on lifestyle changes and come up with techniques to solve memory problems. They can also plan a standard healthcare regimen to control side effects.

- **Head injury:** Some large studies have found that people age 50 or older who have had a traumatic brain injury (TBI) are more likely to develop dementia and Alzheimer's disease. Indeed, the odds are higher in people with more severe and different TBIs. Some things have discovered that opportunity can be most important in the initial six months or two long time after the injury.

- **Discussing Contamination:** Thinking beings have discovered that discussing items of contamination can accelerate the decay of a fearsome frame. People have found that pollution - particularly through reduced activity and wood burning - is associated with a higher risk of dementia.

- **Excessive alcohol consumption:** It has long been known that drinking large amounts of alcohol causes brain changes. Some important considerations and studies have shown that alcohol use disorders have been associated with an increased chance of dementia - early dementia. Prevention Alzheimer's disease is not preventable. In any case, some lifestyle convenience variables can be adjusted. the overall reduction of chances of getting cardiovascular diseases tends to reduce the rate at which one can get dementia. Heart-healthy lifestyle choices to lower your risk of dementia:
- Exercise often

- Eat lean new solid oils and foods like the Mediterranean diet.
- Follow the rules of aftercare to control high blood pressure, diabetes and high cholesterol.
- If you smoke, get help from a doctor to quit smoking. One large, long-term Finnish study found that lifestyle changes helped reduce cognitive decline in people at risk of developing dementia. One-on-one and group sessions were organized for the contemplatives, who focused less on eating, exercising and socializing. In another tired Australian thought, educational sessions were held for people at risk of dementia about eating less, exercising and other lifestyle choices.

changes They performed significantly better on cognitive tests after one, two and three long periods compared to people who did not receive instruction. Other considerations have shown that remaining rationally and socially closed is associated with protected abilities in later life and a lower risk of Alzheimer's disease. This includes participating in social events, going on adventures, exercising, playing board games, art, playing an instrument, and other activities. Inadequate sleep patternsInadequate rest patterns, such as falling asleep or having difficulty falling asleep.

CHAPTER SEVEN.

METHYLENE BLUE FOR AQUACULTURE.

Methylene Blue Application On Fish:

FISH

in this guide, we show in this chapter how methylene blue is used for fish to prevent and treat fungi and other aquatic parasite.

fish are oceanic vertebrates. They typically have gills, compound scales, a long body supported by scales, and are generally cold-blooded."Fish" may be a term used to refer to rays, sharks, coelacanths and ray-finned fishes, but it is not the intended group, which may be a Clade or a group containing a common ancestor and all its relatives Three main classes, groups or types of fish: The hard fish (Osteichthyes), jaw fish (Agnatha) and cartilaginous fish (Chondrichthyes) are the main groups of vertebrates, with more than 33,000 different fish species.No one knows how many different corners there are in the world, but there are always more. Soon we may have over 35,000 or even 40,000 known species! fishes are grouped into three superclasses: the hard fish (Osteichthyes), the jawless fishes (fish), and the cartilaginous angler (Chondrichthyes). Ray-finned fishes are finned fishes in the class, while ray-finned fishes are in the class Sarcopterygii. Both are hard corners. In any case, all fish have some common characteristics that distinguish them from other creatures.

- **Cold-blooded**: All fish are exothermic or cold-blooded, meaning they cannot regulate their internal body temperature. Warm-blooded fish like halibut and mackerel have a type of "regional endothermy," or warm-bloodedness, that is restricted to certain regions.

- **Aquatic Environment:** All fish live in bodies of water, be it fresh or salt water. Be that as it may, not all aquatic animals are anglers.
- **Respiratory gills:** Fish have gills throughout their life cycle. As in the aquatic environment, although all fish have gills, not all animals with gills are gills.
- **Swim bladders:** Specialized organs filled with chatter to keep the angle above water, and in some species help manage mu-oxygen levels. They also provide an additional resting place and are sensitive enough to recognize the development of food and predators.
- **Blades to develop:** The most common are the tail blade, side balances, back blade and butt-focused blade. There are variations, but they all provide mobility, manoeuvrability and strength.

Application Of Methylene Blue On Aquaculture (FISH).

Methylene blue is used in aquaculture as an anti-fungal and anti-parasitic agent and is widely used in the treatment of angler eggs to prevent infectious overgrowth. He manages to kill protozoa and other ocean parasites in the corner.

Methylene blue can be a safe aquarium disinfectant used to treat toxic properties caused by too many smelling salts and nitrites. This mixture is very safe to use and will not harm or kill the fisherman because it is used in limited doses and the fisherman will not overdose.

Period To Apply Methylene Blue For Fish.

Methylene blue is useful against low parasites in the corner. If the angle to be treated is known to be sensitive, this agent is used instead of malachite green to suppress the organisms. MB can be used to prevent infectious diseases in corner eggs and browns. In addition, it is convincing against some external protozoa including Costia, Chilodonella and Ichthyophthirius (Ich)Methylene blue is additionally viable in killing skin and gills, stallions, velvet, organisms and many bacterial diseases and external parasites.

This chemical is very safe to use on many invertebrates. Methylene blue is safe to use with crustaceans such as crabs, shrimp and snails, but should be introduced gradually. It damages living plants, and under such conditions, care must be taken to preserve the plants as they were briefly exposed.

<u>Applying Methylene Blue For Fish.</u>

- **Fish organism Eggs:** The most common purpose of methylene blue in aquaculture is to prevent the development of organisms and microscopic organisms on the surface of eggs. The abundance of parasites and dangerous microscopic organisms around the eggs can cause the eggs to migrate into the aquarium, which can damage the eggs. Methylene blue in this case acts as a disinfectant to fix the recently laid angler eggs. It can additionally help people who wish to misplace corner eggs earlier.

- **Harmful nitrate**: known as "brown blood disease". In this situation, the level of methemoglobin increases, which increases the damage of nitrates. As the nitrate tolerance levels of different marine life forms vary beyond the tolerance limit, the angler becomes diseased and unhealthy as a result of the damage. Broken gills are slow, hang near the water outlets and begin to get a handle on the surface of the water for oxygen, the rapid development of gills is called "kill". Proper use of methylene blue can help eliminate nuisances from tanks.

- **The odour of salts Harmful:** This is caused by an increase in the pH of the tank and affects the nitrogen cycle. This unpleasantness may be due to natural waste or tap water decaying in the tank, but the lack of smelling salt concentration indicates that the water conditions are excellent. Even a small amount of leach damage can be dangerous in breaking angle ends, but large amounts can be much more dangerous to fish survival. Infected fish will gasp for conversation, be drowsy or lethargic, have purple or reddish gills, and blood-red streaks on their bodies and fins, and may spread to the bottom of the tank. Proper use of methylene blue can help eliminate nuisances from tanks.

- **Velvet:** This is also known as odium, rust, or gold cleaning disease. It can be the main common disease of aquarium or aquarium fish. The cause is the parasites Oodinium limnetic and Oodinium, which affect both saltwater and freshwater anglers. fish rub hard surfaces to escape the velvet, but in ambushes, they remain lazy, enter fast and heavy breathing, weight gain, have balance pressed into the body, have lustful need, and rusty or yellow smooth coating. the skin and in extreme cases the skin peels off. In this case, a small amount of "methylene blue" can act as an antiparasitic agent.

- **Thrust:** Anglers regularly strain for a variety of reasons, especially when they are replaced or when conditions in their tank change. In this situation, preventive maintenance is used to relieve the pressure. A dose of "methylene blue" serves as a cover in such a situation.

- **Ick:** This disease is very similar to skin contamination. Contaminated fish will start clawing at rocks and stones and may become lethargic as they progress. Such pollution makes the skin modest white spots that take sand, as well as blood-red streaks or redness in conditions of extensive pollution.

- **Swim bladder confusion:** This is caused by a swim bladder that is not functioning properly. Its usability can be affected by mechanical or natural components such as infection or physical imperfection. Dirty corners seem to have many side effects such as sinking to the bottom of the aquarium, struggling to maintain your position and standing on your head, landing upside down and problems with buoyancy. They have a bent back or a bulging stomach, so their physical appearance is also somehow affected. Methylene blue is also convincing in the treatment of this condition.

How To Utilize Methylene Blue For Fish.

When your fish's life is in danger, choosing the right medication can be a critical and intense choice. Consider making an intensive list of all the inhabitants of your aquarium that have recently sought care.

- Note the recommendations on product packages or the advice of a nearby corner manager, sometimes recently added to the methylene blue container.
- For coordinated aquarium use, a general rule of thumb is 1 drop of liquid methylene blue or 1 teaspoon of powder mixture per 10 gallons of water. To prepare a seawater solution for a saltwater angle, combine 1 teaspoon of the drug with 5 litres of water. Do not put the methylene blue powder directly into the container or crush it into a

small amount of water and then mix it into the container.

- Add 1 teaspoon of 2.303% methylene blue to 10 litres of water to prevent or treat organisms in fish eggs. This occurs at a concentration of 3 ppm. Higher concentrations usually include 1/3 teaspoon (1.64 ml) per 10 gallons for every 1 ppm increase.

- As if one application were needed. Treatment should be resumed 3 days after free swimming or 2 days after delivery of live carriers.

- Methylene blue can also be used to treat parasitic infections, fish infected with external protozoan parasites or fish suffering from cyanide damage.

- Design a non-metallic holder large enough to hold the corner machined while filling it with water from the starting tank.

- Add 5 tablespoons (24.65 ml) for every 3 litres of water. This occurs at a concentration of 50 ppm. It is not recommended to extend the concentration above 50 ppm.

- Immerse the workpiece in this arrangement for a maximum of 10 seconds.
- Re-enable angular in a unique container.

Safety Measures In Using Methylene Blue For Fish Treatment.

Below are some steps to take when using methylene blue in fish processing.

- Under certain conditions, processing most tanks is an alternative to solve the problem. If you use MB, you should treat your important tank specifically to improve chemically toxic properties or fight external parasites. In this situation, driving out the living carbon channel to protect the microscopic organisms inside is very important, and you push it away.

- Methylene blue can be a powerful phytotoxin, meaning it targets all kinds of microscopic organisms and microorganisms, even beneficial organisms and microorganisms. Usually one of the most common reasons why dosing an aquarium instead of a separate tank is dangerous. If you have recently showered or taken medication, move your corner to a temporary storage container.

- Methylene blue should not be used at the same time as erythromycin or tetracycline.

- After using methylene blue, monitor your tank just as you would with any other treatment. After three to five days, usually replace a quarter of the water in your aquarium and carbon channel.

CHAPTER EIGHT.

METHYLENE BLUE DOSAGE AND SIDE EFFECTS.

Most Prescribed Dose For Methylene Blue.

Based on the studies and research done, we can say that methylene blue is dosed at 0.045-0.09 ml per kilogram of body weight. In exceptional cases, administer methylene blue (methylene blue infusion) intravenously gradually over several minutes.

What Drugs, Substances, Or Supplements Associated With Methylene Blue:

Methylene blue can be associated with acetazolamide, laxatives, sodium bicarbonate or diuretics (water pills). Tell your expert about all your solutions.

Methylene Blue Amid Pregnancy Or Breastfeeding.

Methylene blue can harm the baby, but this drug can sometimes be used during pregnancy. Your specialist will decide whether this medicine is safe or not. Tell your specialist if you are pregnant. It is not known whether methylene blue passes into the chest drain or if it could harm a nursing baby. Consult your specialist during recent breastfeeding.

Side Effects Of Methylene Blue:

Some of the side effects of using methylene blue include:

- loose bowels
- difficulty breathing
- difficulty swallowing
- irregular heart rate
- rapid heart rate
- fever

- brain pain
- hives or swelling, tingling or rash on the skin
- expanding, bee-like swelling of the face, eyelids, lips, tongue, throat, hands, feet, legs or genitals
- overactive reflexes
- pale skin
- poor coordination
- fast pulse
- flushing of the skin
- irritability
- tremors
- sore throat
- sweating
- crazy talking or behaviour that you cannot control
- tremors or shaking
- twitching
- bluish lips, fingernails or palms
- chest pain
- alarm
- hacker

- boring pee.

<u>Symptoms Of Overdose In Using Methylene Blue.</u>

if you overdose or fail to follow the prescription of a doctor or healthcare provider under any of the main symptoms:

- confusion
- cloudy urine
- difficulty breathing
- tiredness or unsteadiness
- unsteadiness, fainting, or unsteadiness. suddenly lying down or sitting up
- fear
- fever
- migraine
- anger
- pale skin
- rapid pulse
- rapid shallow breathing
- sore throat
- abdominal pain
- abnormal death or bruising

- strange tiredness or weakness
- swaying

General Dosage:

This guide does not provide a specific dosage of methylene blue, it is best advised to follow the physician's description when choosing to use methylene blue solution.

THE END.

www.ingramcontent.com/pod-product-compliance
Lightning Source LLC
Chambersburg PA
CBHW050811250726
48653CB00006B/2159